THINK LIKE A
SKINNY PERSON

James Livingood

FORWARD

After failing at my weight loss New Years resolutions time and time again, I decided to change things up. The idea was to ask my skinny friends what they thought of food and exercise. I thought that maybe I would lose 2-3 lbs. I ended up losing 75 lbs. **The way that these skinny people thought had a tremendous effect in my life!**

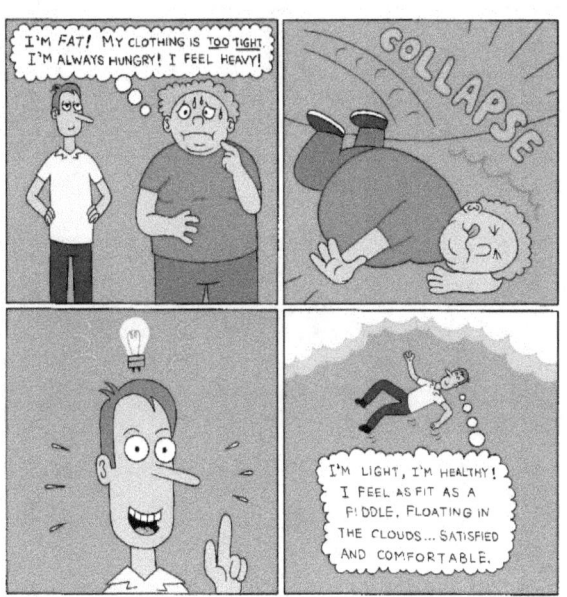

No one tip made this happen.

(I also continue to add new tips here: www.thinklikeaskinnyperson.com)

Instead it was a collection of tips and advice, which I am going to share here in this book. However, before I begin: **THANK YOU** Jeb, Shanail, Cory, and Erin/Joe V!

Not only for answering my questions, but for being there for me. Thank you!

INTRODUCTION

I am in love with bullet points. Automatic numbering drives me wild. Italics, bold, underlined - I can't get enough. As far back as I can remember, I have been list oriented. Perhaps these lists help me feel in control, or perhaps they make it easy to review my thoughts, but either way - I am a fan of making lists.

So it was with much frustration that during my 10 year New Years resolution review (sadly, not a joke) I found a trend. Two themes kept appearing: better finances and better health. The finances had steadily improved, but the health had slowly grown worse. I decided that the problem was not finding the one perfect solution. Instead, I needed to find out what I didn't know.

I decided to build a list. This list would include a bunch of tips from my skinny friends. The idea was that if I had enough of these tips I would see a trend and know how to "Think Like a Skinny Person". With any luck, I would not only lose a few pounds, but would be on track to keep them off. I ended up losing 75 pounds. While that may not fully qualify me as skinny, I did have a lot of people asking what I did.

For most of us, our brains resemble an episode of "Hoarders". In that TV show, people collect a bunch of small bits of junk in the hope that one day a piece will be used. All of our past experiences with dieting and exercise may have resulted in a heap of mental trash. A fad diet or food failed us, but we hold onto the experience as some kind of evidence.

I've included some questions, tips, and cartoons along the way to keep you motivated. There is a lot of work to do! The more you interact the better. Disagree, agree, think of another solution, whatever: so long as you interact.

Please note that I am not a health care expert and have no formal education in nutrition. I simply know what has worked for me and want to share that knowledge.

PART ONE

Know Yourself

"What gets measured gets managed" - Peter Drucker.

The first part of this book is not about giving you a bunch of advice. Instead we will take a moment to look into the mirror. Understanding and planning, while going hand-in-hand, are often exclusive. We understand that decreasing calories and increasing exercise will output more energy. The higher the energy output, the more weight we will lose. However, we don't build plans enough to help facilitate this goal.

Here is the difference:

1.) I want to look good

2.) I want to fit a size ##, which requires me to lose 30 lbs. Each pound is 3500 calories. I want to fit into this garment by summer, which is three months away.

That means 10 lbs per month which breaks down to 1166 calories per 30 days. - Now how can I cut that amount of calories per my daily diet (and still be healthy)?

It should be obvious which one of those two paths is more likely to lead to action. Steps still need to be created for both, but the approach is very different.

Know your Timing

Knowing your eating habits is also an important step towards building a plan of action. Does this mostly happen late at night? Do you skip breakfast? Do you only eat when the kids eat? By knowing these particular timing habits, you can begin to build a pattern. Once you have a pattern established, you have points at which you can measure. For example, if you eat more in the evening after stressful day at work, you have a crucial measurement point. Did you stress eat today after work? Or did you read a post-it note on the fridge and then went for a quick walk right after work? How did you handle coming home after work?

Beyond knowing these crucial daily timings, there are weekly and monthly events that happen. Holidays often mess with our timing more than we like to admit. Holidays are more than just the major events. Vacations, birthdays, office parties, etc are all special events which mess up our food timings. If we don't have a plan for these events in advance, we are more likely to fail.

One of the most popular excuses during holidays is that the event is "special" which gives a person a pass to eat junk. After all, Christmas comes only once a year right? Easter comes but once a year, St. Patrick's Day, Valentines, Thanksgiving, 4th of July, person X's birthday, person Y's birthday, your own birthday, your significant other's birthday, the summer beach trip, the spring vacation, favorite TV show, the road trip in the late summer, popcorn at the theater, the pumpkin patch, the office party, Halloween, on and on and on. There is always some special event going on. Having a plan for these events is crucial because special events happen a lot. These events should not have a free pass to modify our goals. Part of identifying the timing of how we eat is in identifying the unique circumstance that derail our progress.

When special is not so special

Many of these unique events have custom foods. The pressure to eat these foods comes from the false idea of scarcity. While a sugar cookie in the shape of a pumpkin may appear like a "limited time only" deal, is that true? In less than a month there will be sugar cookies in the shape of a tree. Both cookies taste the same, only the shape is different. Seeing as these cookies are essentially the same, do we have to eat the cookie now? Or can we wait a few months? It is essentially the same cookie, so any scarcity is a lie. Not only could we get this same cookie later, we could even produce the cookie at our desire. There is nothing stopping a person from making Christmas cookies in July. There is not some unique harvested ingredient that is only available for use in December.

Let's expand this concept further: eating when sad and glad. There is a deadly cycle when food becomes intertwined between these two emotions. As we talked about, we like to eat special foods to celebrate. A vacation or holiday may see us eating more than normal. We give ourselves a pass to eat poorly because we want to enhance our happiness at that moment. Feasting to celebrate is a custom that follows us far into the past. We get together and eat well to show joy. The problem with this feasting is that there becomes an urge to constantly feast. Instead of a once a year event or once-in-a-lifetime event, we end up eating a bunch throughout the month. Perhaps it is Friday and a person wants to celebrate the weekend? Perhaps we are going to a restaurant with friends on Saturday? Perhaps we want to eat a bunch during a Sunday sporting event? Feasting to show joy creeps into more and more of our lives. The rarity of the events continues to less more and more, until we start celebrating anything.

So when happens when we have a bad day? Work doesn't go well, or there is some financial stress keeping us down. We may not want to worry about doing the dishes, so we pick up some quick junk food. Much like joy eating above, this type of sad eating may start out as occasional. However, soon the events shift from major to minor. Instead of eating as a way to cope from losing your job, you eat because work ran 30 minutes late. Instead of eating because you had a major argument with a family member, your stress eating because the family event has awkward silences.

The truly insidious thing about celebration feasting and sad eating, is that they work so well together. A person that eats to celebrate good times is much more likely to eat to cope with bad times. As discussed above, the level of good and bad relaxes over time. Given enough time a person may start to binge eat, not because of a good / bad event, but because ANY event happened. The same can be true of other coping mechanisms such as drinking. Realizing a bird's eye perspective may help detach this level of sad and glad eating. The only consistent thing in this life is change. Nothing you eat will stop change from happening. So instead of trying to "enhance" the moment or "skip past" the moment, be present. Don't try to relive a memory by eating junk food. Don't try to hide an emotion by ordering extra French fries. Instead learn to separate out food from mood and build a better perspective.

In the mood for a craving

We all get in the mood for a unique food from time to time. We call these moods cravings, and attach to them the stigma that they won't be satisfied until we eat what we are longing for. The truth behind cravings is that there are two different types and that we are often bad distinguishing between them. A false craving is one where we see an object and want that object now. Once we no longer see that object, the desire slips from our minds and onto other things. A true craving is one where we desire an object and continue to do so, long after it has slipped our viewpoint.

A great example of true and false cravings are impulse items at the checkout stand. We may not have realized how much we want a candy bar until we get there. However, if we ignore this candy and walk out the store, we no longer want that candy bar. This candy bar impulse item is a great example of a false craving. If a person were truly craving a candy bar, they would have picked it up long before the checkout lane. Furthermore, they would go back into the store to purchase the item. Understanding the difference between these two is important. Once a person can identify true and false cravings, they can remove a lot of the power junk food has over us. Instead of needing the junk food at a moment, they learn to wait and destroy the craving. Furthermore, by understanding a true craving, they don't buy into all the extras. Instead of buying a bunch of stuff to go "along with" the craving, they just buy the single item. This leads to better caloric control. So instead of buying fries with that burger and a shake too, they just buy the burger. Furthermore, true cravings have higher amounts of satisfaction associated with them. Often times a person will go without to understand if the craving is true or not. When they realize that the craving is true, they savor the food more. It is no longer a quick "means to an end". They are no longer buying the food just to scratch a quick itch. People that do scratch every craving itch (true or false) end up with more cravings. This constant scratching is one way that non-stop snacking starts to happen.

Hunger is not an emergency

One of the best ways to determine if a craving is true or false is to wait. The same is true about hunger. Hunger is not an emergency that needs to be solved immediately. Unless there are problems with blood sugar, hunger is rarely an emergency. Feeling slight discomfort in your stomach is not a huge problem. To put this into focus, eating to avoid hunger is like constantly spreading on a layer of pain relieving ointment. After enough time, we become overly sensitized to the feeling, and start avoiding small discomfort at all costs. Not only does this over sensitization rob us of our focus, it takes a lot of energy and time. Being a little hungry is OK and can even help us appreciate our food later on. That being said, being hungry does not give us a pass to binge eat later.

Too much of anything, even good things, can quickly turn bad. Drinking too much water can kill. Eating too much salad and leave a body deficient in specific nutrients. Over exercise can have long term effects on our muscular skeletal systems. Moderation is the key to success in many areas. Even behaving properly should be in moderation. The point of existing isn't to leave by leading a near perfect life.

PART TWO

Stress

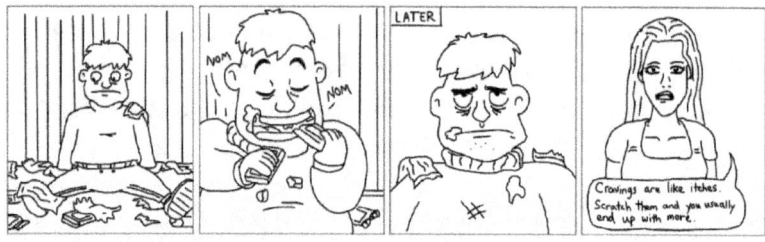

Stress eating is a tricky and complex problem. Most often stress eating is a kind of self medication to get you through the day. Here are some questions to see if you have stress eating problems:

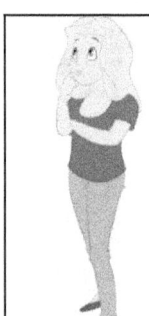

Q1: Do you look forward to ending the day eating in front of the TV?

Q2: Do you buy a lot of fast food during bad days?

Q3: Do you have secret stashes of food?

Everybody experiences some sort of worry or anxiety. Some wear their emotions on their sleeves, while others keep them buried within. Those that bury their stress tend to have much more difficulty. Either way, we need to recognize and deal with those emotions. If we don't work through the emotions, we will succumb to them. Situations can not be wished away. They require focus and removing that which obstructs a person. A person must rise above their anxiety, not sink below.

One thing that a person must do when their starting to learn to manage stress is learn to not be so critical. No one is perfect and everyone has difficult times in their life. However, having those troublesome times is not an excuse to eat unhealthy. We all have stress, even skinny people. The best way to understand how to deal with unhealthy stress is to recognize the emotions around food. By knowing when emotions happen, the more likely we are to deal with them. A person can learn what it takes to eat healthy, under stressful circumstances. This technique is a very tricky thing for many people to do. The idea of comfort food is based around the negating of a person's emotions with junk food. This section will teach how to recognize stress levels.

Signs of stress

The first thing we want to talk about is recognizing emotions. There are two different ways to recognize emotions. The first is to find internal markers while the second is to use external markers. Seeing these different markers can help a person realize that it is time to start working on their stress levels.

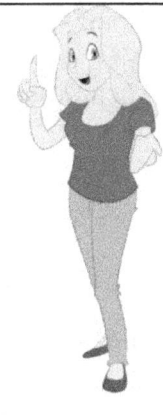

Stress Markers

- Many people identify stress with the purely physical markers.
- Pulse speeds up
- Sweating a lot
- Icy like sensation
- Muscles going tight, sometimes involuntarily
- Breath gets heavier
- Stomach feels pitted out
- Needing to go the bathroom a lot
- Even strong people feel exhausted
- Can't think clearly and make decisions
- A person becomes impartial to things they were passionate about
- A person feels remorseful
- A person feels terrible, even about the simple things
- A person may be irritable
- Some even get the giggles

If stress continues into the long haul, changes may become truly radical. A person may eat a lot or sleep more than regular. Some may smoke, gamble, and drink more. Some may disregard social connections, such as work and friends. Others may let their looks go or get extra clingy around others. People with constant stress may be very negative with everything they have to say. So what are some markers can can be used to determine stress, beyond high pulse rates and heavy breathing?

Internal markers are those within a person. Anger anxiety tends to have many internal markers. Some people eat when they are angry, while others scream. A person can determine if they have anger anxiety by using two different signs. The first sign of anger is if they are raising their voice. The second sign of anger is if they start to throw things or flail their arms around a lot. These are internal symptoms that can show a person's true feelings. These symptoms typically surface during stressful periods.

On the opposite side of anger is depression anxiety. There are many symptoms with depression. Everyone has a depressing time in their life. However if a person is having constant depression, that may require medical help. Some symptoms of depression include talking in a very quiet voice, shying away from social situations, or sleeping a lot more than normal. These events show an internal emotion of depression. Depression is also a common indication of stress.

This second set of markers are very external. Many people will only use internal markers to discover stress, but external ones are equally as useful. Some external markers include watching too much TV, playing to many video games, or watching a lot of movies. Other external symptoms may also be surfing the web too much. A drastic shift in fashion can also be an external sign of stress (suddenly wearing a lot of sweat pants). Music preference can also be a great indication of stress levels. These external signs can help show stress, even if the internal signs appear fine. Keeping an eye on routine habits (such as TV, music, movies, and Internet) can help a person discover if their under a lot of stress.

However you identify stress, there is no doubt it has a negative impact on the body. Our body is a power that we control and can build the experience we want in life. We are not meant to flounder in anxiety and do nothing about it. Our minds and bodies are equipped to find ways to deal with these anxieties, we simply have to unlock them. Many times we feel as though we can't get past tough times. Perhaps we agonize of choices we've made in life. The reality is that stress is a highlighter. Stress and anxiety are only meant to show us where to focus efforts and are not meant to defeat us. Building this focus means being a champ at fighting these internal battles.

Decrease Stress Eating

Now that stress has been identified, we will work through some basic motions on removing stress eating. We will then move into defusing stress at work and relationships. By removing this stress, we can gain power in our everyday actions. With luck, this power will help build momentum toward the correct actions.

Anxiety Eating

The first motion to be described is angry or anxiety stress eating. There are several different ways to understand the emotion. More often then not this habit is a form of self medicating. We feel bad about something in our lives and want endorphins in our head. These endorphins are released by junk and comfort foods. By re-framing the action as "self-medicating" much of the power is taken away. Another way to frame this type of eating is understanding Pavlov's dog.

Pavlov trained his dog to drool on command. This action was completed by ringing a bell every time the dog got a treat. Soon, treat or not, the dog would start drooling when the bell rang. We humans also act in a very simple manner. Watching for this behavior can be a key to re-directing the energy. For example, if a person always eats during commercials or at a specific time every day. Habit can become a powerful force, for better or worse.

A final idea on removing anxiety stress eating is to trade out the behavior. Many skinny people will use exercise or other positive behaviors to work out their anxiety. Completing exercise not only curbs anxiety and angry, but decreases calories and sends a similar endorphin to the brain (via runner's high).

Depressed Eating

The second major motion to be described is depressed eating. This behavior is probably the largest bad habit not talked about. Furthermore, when combined with television, this behavior becomes extra insidious. We get bored with what we are watching, so we look for something new or novel, which is often the food in the fridge. When depressed we cling to any little bit to fun to be had, and that includes TV / food. We need to instead recognize that the brain shuts down when depressed. To help curb and remove depression, the brain needs a challenge. This can be done through changing the scenery or trying out a new adventure. Having social time is also extremely important. However, these ideas will only work for mild to mid depression. Clinical, long term depression may require a medical professional to help. They are armed with more tools and techniques than can be fit into this book.

A great tip to help combat depressed eating is to go to bed early or to change out the routine. Cleaning instead of raiding the fridge works well. Building events that a person looks forward to is also a great way to combat depression. When a person is excited to go to an event, they are less likely to eat a massive amount of calories. Instead, a person may be saving calories for that special event. Furthermore, they may be regulating their mental health to be prepared for that upcoming event.

Decrease Overall Stress

Here are several routines that can work the worry from a person's life. Executing these tips would may help renew a person's lease on life.

Relax

One of the hardest muscles to relax is a person's mind. The mind obstructs positive reactions from your body. To counter that, deep breathing activities can work in an incredible fashion. Take a seat, and breathe in deeply. Released the air slowly from the lungs. Concentrate on removing thoughts and just focus on the breathing.

Acknowledge the Stress

Sometimes the best step to defeat stress is to admit how much stress a person is under. Once discovered, a person can being to work on the problems. This insight is an essential step towards the removal of stress. Categorizing stress will also help to dissipate the anxiety.

Talk with People You Trust

After the stress is acknowledged, talk to a trusted friend or family member. The more respectable their opinion, the better. Who is the one you believe the most? Let them know your issues. You will find that offering your issue dependably makes it lighter. Even if they can't help, sometimes knowing that they are thinking of you helps decrease a person's stress.

Look for Your Fun and Relaxation

Invest time with a pastime. On the off chance that a person likes viewing films, do that activity. In the event that a person would rather twist up with a book, do that. Sometimes having some fun in a favorite activity, even just a brief moment, can work wonders. Sometimes reviewing old silly photos or re-living silly actions can help snap us out of a funk. If a person really enjoyed an old video game in their youth, playing that game may gain a new insight. If a person hasn't seen the face of the high school friends for a long time, perhaps a yearbook will help spark some perspective.

Don't Lose the Humor

Regardless of the fact that what is happening is causing anxiety, it doesn't imply that you ought to turn grouchy and crotchety. Bear in mind how to snicker. Watch some great drama shows or read some clever books or simply stick around with your companions who like to tell jokes. Pursue and study humor, as that action can help break a sour mood caused by anxiety and stress.

Decrease Work Stress

Work and stress are often synonyms. We spend so much time at work that there is no wonder on why the activity is so stressful. Here are several quick tips to remove stress at work.

Learn to say no if the work is too much. Understanding that poor work can be worse then no work is one way to curb this behavior. Furthermore, helping establishing boundaries helps other as well. By knowing exactly what they can expect, a co-worker will use the work relationship in a more accurate manner. Many people keep piling on work because they are afraid to establish boundaries with clients and co-workers. However, these boundaries are what help the work maintain its quality. Adding more work on top will lead to poor quality work.

Another method do decrease work stress is to be pro-active. Many times individuals will only acknowledge due dates that are immediate or come with a threat. Instead, look for upcoming deadlines and combat those. By having deadlines done in advance, less worry needs to happens. This worry often is decreased because as unforeseen events happen, time is built in to help mitigate those circumstances. When a deadline is due immediately, and an unforeseen event happens, stress can skyrocket.

Prioritizing is a topic with many different methods of approach. Some believe that a person should complete their least favorite task first. Others believe that simple tasks should be taken care of immediately, moderate tasks scheduled, and hard tasks broken off / delegated. Some people believe that having post-it notes around the monitor helps warn a person. Others believe that Outlook reminders are the way to go. Whatever method is used for prioritizing, I would recommend experimenting and finding what works well for your situation. While many methods will not work, finding a workable solution is a huge success. For myself, this includes completing tasks in a single shot. Sitting down and working on the task until it is completely finished.

Take time for education. Many disregard the importance of learning new things at work. Not only does making time for learning help decrease the stress, but it can help a person from feeling they are falling behind the curve. This education can be as formal as a certification program or as informal as a YouTube video. Either way, making time for education at work is important.

Take time for friends and family. One of the biggest work stresses is feeling like the connection to loved ones is strained. While less time may be available, making time for quality connections is important. By maintaining this connection, people will feel less guilty and therefore less stressed about work. Lunch with work companions can also help to serve this function. One interesting perspective is to celebrate work achievements with non-work family and companions. While this action may feel vain, brining family and friends into the celebration helps them feel connected to your work. They feel part of your success, which helps them understand why you may work extra hard.

Work and stress are words that can often be switched for each other. However, this stress doesn't have to have such a negative or evil connotation. Dealing with these stress triggers allows a person to convert work stress to a positive motivating factor.

Decrease Relationship Stress

Many relationships come with a complex type of anxiety. As we reveal truths about ourselves to others, what we find is often uncomfortable and difficult. Here are several methods to decrease relationship anxiety.

Sometimes the quickest way to decrease stress is to realize that everyone is human. Being human means that each and everyone of us is imperfect in some way. Understanding and forgiving yourself for imperfections is an important first step in dealing with relationship stress. Furthermore, a party should not be put on a pedestal and worshiped (or vice versa).

Another idea to decrease stress is to focus on why the relationship exists. What specifically does the relationship solve? The reason needs to be significant. If a relationship exists just to be fun and exciting, that is a recipe for trouble. No relationship maintains fun and excitement forever, which can then cause stress. Uncovering motivation will help ensure that no ulterior thought process is going on.

Another way to decrease stress it to accept a person's faults. Trying to change a behavior or appearance can cause stress and decrease desire. Many individuals are changed away from the traits that originally scored them the relationship. When this happens, a person no longer feel attracted and leaves. This leaves the abandoned party feeling clueless and responsible. The truth is that the other party may be to blame.

A helpful idea to avoid relationship stress is to work towards de-identifying. Many times we build exclusions for our paramours. They are given free passes because we care for them. If they were put in a de-identified role (them vs a generic companion/mate) we would see those special exclusions we give them. Often times understanding these exclusions can help build boundaries, which can decrease stress.

Also make sure to make time, both when required and not. Not only will this help maintain the health of the relationship, but it will keep many of the negative stress arguments out of the relationship.

Don't keep privileged insights. Being open about potential pot holes and problems is key to resolving them quickly. Being silent on these problems can lead to additional stress and worry later on. At the same time, remember that your both human and both full of flaws.

Yet another great tip is to discuss the association between the two of you. One may believe that a relationship is deeper than the other may believe. Talking about these differences allows a more even playing field. The better the playing field, the less stress for both parties involved.

Practice random surprises of love. Showing that you care, when they don't expect it, is a great way to relieve stress. This type of act sets the precedent that even when away, your thinking of them. Many times we think the worst case scenario, when the opposite is true. By having a precedent of random acts of love, a relationship has a better ground to stand on.

Remember that a relationship is a function between two people. Understanding why people need that connection is the first step to nurturing that connection.

Once a person understands their stance in a relationship they feel less stress.

Stress, boredom, anxiety, angry, and many other emotions force us to eat more than we should. These emotions lead to a lot of junk food decisions. No one is perfect, so understanding these emotions is a way we can forgive ourselves. Furthermore we give ourselves permissions to quickly recover from an occasional mess up. By learning to deal with individual emotions, we build a better self control. The more self control we have, the better relationship we have with food. This is what "Think Like a Skinny Person" is all about: building a better relationship with food.

PART THREE

Sleep

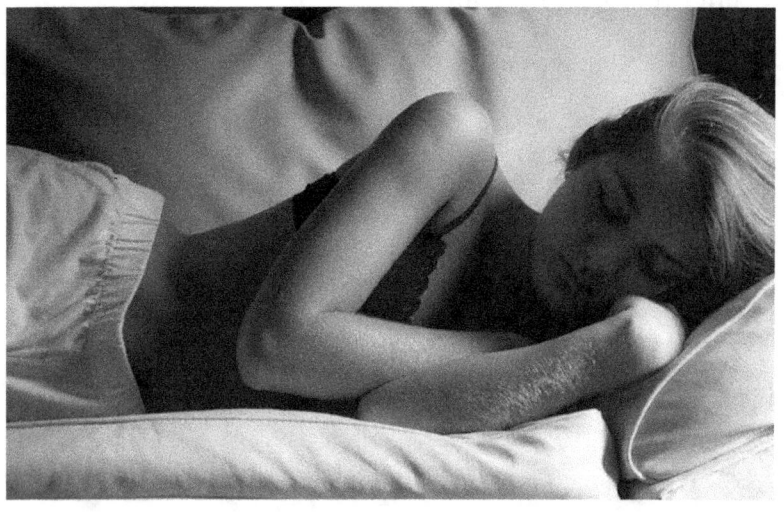

Sleep is a vital part of great health. Here are some questions to see if you are getting enough sleep.

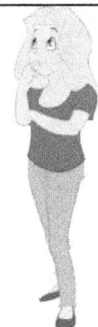

Q1: Do you wake up sore?

Q2: Do you wake up multiple times during the night?

Q3: Did you spend a good amount on your mattress?

Sleep is a very important topic for skinny people. These people know that having a restful night today is important toward having a fantastic day tomorrow. Sleep allows a mental refresh as well as a refresh from exercise. Having a mental refresh enhances a person's productivity and creativity the next day. They use this mental boost to help them discover new exercise routines and diet choices. Some skinny people even use sleep as a way to avoid eating after dinner. Skinny people know that cravings after dinner can be squashed with going to bed early. This method is a surefire way to keep the calories down. Those that stay awake too long suffer from increased calories as well as other mental problems.

When a weekday hour is not equal to a weekend hour.

So why do we stay up so late? Beyond that we are exceedingly busy, it is natural for our minds to slowly stay up progressively later. Skipping out on sleep for a few days in a row doesn't feel like a cumulative effect.

However, we don't fully take into consideration the way sleep helps our bodies.

Our digestive system, nervous system, and muscle systems need regular sleep. When we deprive our brains of sleep, we also deprive these individual systems repair time. Tests have shown that lab rats, who receive regular sleep deprivation, have shorter life expectancy.

If we start a deficit on the weekday, some of those hours can be made up on the weekend. What most people don't realize, is that not all of this deficit can be made up.

This "sleep debt" can lead to impaired vision, raised blood pressure, insulin resistance, weight gain, and cardiac problems. Our bodies are not meant to have any sleep debt, especially not continual debt that needs to be repaid. To gain a better understanding on paying sleeping debt, one hour asleep on the weekend is not worth four hours skipped over the week. Instead research suggests that all four hours must be made up. Here is the very deadly part of "sleep debt"; the body can only do so many sleep rhythms per night. That means there is a ceiling on how much "sleep debt" a person has before it carries over.

The amount of sleep required to repair changes depending on several factors. Pregnant women require more sleep than their non-pregnant counterparts. Furthermore, children may need more sleep than adults. A typical adult requires 7-9 hours of sleep every night.

Internal Signs of Sleep Deprivation

One of the most obvious signs are micro naps. These are instances where a person loses consciousness for a short period of time. These people may not even realized that they were asleep. Many deaths on the road are attributed to micro naps.

Constant yawning and an inability to focus are also signs of being tired. Beyond being able to focus, tired people have trouble remembering facts as well. There is an irony for many sleep deprived. That irony is that they stay up late trying to work but do a much worse the next work day.

Lacking motivation and depression are additional symptoms of sleep deprivation. When a person's mind is shutting down, these are common symptoms. While an mentally engaged person can have these symptoms too, they are much more likely in a person with sleep deprivation.

Spotting Sleep Deprivation in Others

One way to measure if a person is sleep deprived is to see how much television they are watching. Sleep deprived people will be less specific about what they are watching. Instead they will channel surf or simply continue watching the same channel. For example, if their favorite show plays, they will watch the next one and the one after that. They may not truly want to watch these shows, but their mind is tired enough that the mind simply accepts these as the next regular step.

Another external sign of sleep deprivation is if a person keeps re-reading the same sentence. They may also keep re-reading the same paragraph. The mind wants to continue reading, but is no longer able to absorb anymore with adequate sleep.

If a person is playing video games, their character may keep "running into walls". This behavior is because they are nodding off while playing the video game.

Another indication of being tired is an observation on posture. If a person starts out straight in a chair, and slowly slumps overtime, you can tell they are getting ready for bed. Some people will even, without knowing it, make the couch or chair into a bed. They start slumping, then put on a blanket, add some pillows... and start sleeping! Instead they should simply go to bed early and get more restful sleep. Sleeping in chairs and couches is a great way to wake up with a knot in your neck or back.

Yet another sign a person is tired is in how they interact with others. During the start of the night, a person may be more talkative. As the night continues on, topics may become simpler or they may stop talking entirely. These people are getting more and more mentally sleepy, and can therefore use less and less of this complex part of their brain. The same is true for other forms of social communication. These include social networks, text messages, and phone calls. As a person becomes sleepier and sleepier, their communications get simpler. Furthermore, spelling errors and grammar problems may creep into their communication.

One final way to tell if a person is tired is to check with their devices. Many devices only hold a day or less of charge. If the device has had a lot of use, and is almost out of power, then a person can know it is time for bed. Not only can these tablets, smart phones, and laptops recharge overnight, but their owners can too.

Improving Sleep - Physical Tricks

The best way to improve sleep is to have more sleep. For many of us, that may be difficult or not as important. Perhaps a person keeps waking up in the middle of the night. Perhaps a person wakes up stiff and sore in the morning. Sometimes having more sleep is only the beginning. Here are several methods for improving sleep.

We spend so much time in our beds. However, people underestimate how much money they spend on a bed. Getting a great bed is the best first step towards a better nights sleep. Getting quality pillows and blankets are another fantastic idea. A person spends so much time sleeping in their bed that it only makes sense. Furthermore, a great bed can lead to deep and more rejuvenating sleep. This deeper sleep can have a big affect on the upcoming day.

Another way to improve sleep is to build a regular sleep cycle. Going to bed at the same time every night has some interesting benefits. The biggest benefit is that the mind undergoes Pavlov's response. Pavlov was a scientist who trained his dogs with a bell. Every time he rung the bell, the dogs got a treat. Getting these treats made the dogs drool. Soon, Pavlov took the treats away. What he discovered was that the dogs began to drool whenever the bell was rung, even when no treats are available. This experiment shows the power of mental training.

When the mind goes to sleep at a regular time, when that time comes, the mind puts itself to sleep. This means that insomnia and other negative symptoms are avoided. In addition to this, waking up at the same time helps the mind feel more awake quicker. That means that less needs to be done to convince the mind to start working.

Avoiding liquids and caffeine at night are also good ways to get a restful night sleep. Avoiding liquids ensures that a person will not have to pee during the night. Caffeine can also trick the brain into being more away then it should. Having too much food can also cause a stomach ache that can keep a person up. There are also some mental tricks to help a person go to sleep.

Improving Sleep - Mental Tricks

One of the most common old trick is counting sheep. This can work because the mind focuses on the task instead of the events of the day. Ultimately, this method is how a person can go to bed. There are a few other tricks a person can do.

Lighting and heat are two common factors that a person can use to put their mind in the mood for sleep. Low or no light can help convince the mind to sleep. Furthermore, some people enjoy a warm or cold room when going to sleep.

Another common trick is to try and mentally focus on "thinking nothing". As a person keeps striving toward doing this, they start falling more and more asleep. The trick with this method is to keep reminding yourself to not think about anything. The mind will naturally want to recap the day. Recent television shows, work schedules, and conversations should be purged from the mind. This method is much like counting sheep, but is a new spin on an old classic. Thinking nothing to some people may be a white canvas, while others may view this as a black canvas. What happens is that the mind eventually relaxes and then converts into dreams. A person will lose control of "thinking nothing" when they sleep.

People also work toward this "thinking nothing" trick by using a few other methods. One method is to put some distance between highly mental, engaging activities and sleep. For example, instead of playing an exciting video game before bed, they read. Reading may not be as exciting as constant action and sound. Additional lights and sounds may be removed from the bedroom as well. This reduction can include clocks, television sets, and computer screens. The idea is to remove as many mental stimulations as possible, reducing activities to those less stimulating. Doing this reduction on a regular basis is a great way to ensure fantastic sleep.

Finally, those that suffer from insomnia on a regular basis need to build "cut off" points. Many people with insomnia will stay up much longer then they want. Instead, when it starts getting too late, they need to take some sleep medication. Being stubborn is not a good idea when having insomnia. Sleep medication will lead to a less restful night, but can be helpful if insomnia is driving a person up too late. Constant insomnia is also a reason to seek medical attention. There may be a medication or other condition causing the insomnia.

Power Naps

Sometimes the best way to pay a sleep debt, or to simple be more mentally capable, is to have a power nap. If your workplace is one of the few places that offers a sleep space, make use of it. However, many people don't have work environments that encourage this kind of behavior. Instead they can do the following tips.

Taking a 10-minute nap in a car during a break or during lunch can be quite restful. The trick with this method is to ensure that distractions are minimized. Furthermore, it may be best to avoid other staff from seeing this, as they will believe you are over-tired. A person may not be over-tired to take a nap. They may simply want to be more productive in their daily lives. If the car is not available, it may be possible to take a nap in an office. Office naps require locking the door and making sure no one interrupts. These are often the most difficult to pull off, as people have trouble understanding why they can't contact you.

Another great way to enhance a power nap is to workout earlier in the day. By nap time the body will be more ready to sleep. Oxygen levels in the blood will be better as well as overall drowsiness and fatigue. Sleep and exercise patterns can greatly influence each other.

Eating a lunch that is not high in sugar and carbohydrates is a way to encourage good power naps. Lower fat proteins can help blood sugar and make energy last. While people may assume that high carbohydrates would lead to good power naps, the truth is that these power naps are often highly erratic (waking up a lot). The best method to enter a power nap is to not have blood sugar influencing the brain.

Learning to meditate is also a great way to enter into a power nap. Meditation helps reduce the "noise" of the day. This reduction of noise helps focus towards regular sleeping. Breathing meditation (focusing only on breaths) is an excellent way to start a great power nap.

Skinny people are aware of not only what they eat, but how they feel. When they are sleepy, they don't fight their bodies to stay up extra late. Instead they know that a successful day tomorrow starts with a good night beforehand. This restful night leads to more bodily repair as well as mental focus. Skinny people also have more motivation in their following day when they had a great night's sleep beforehand. Few things on TV can compete with the benefits of a great night's sleep.

PART FOUR

Workout

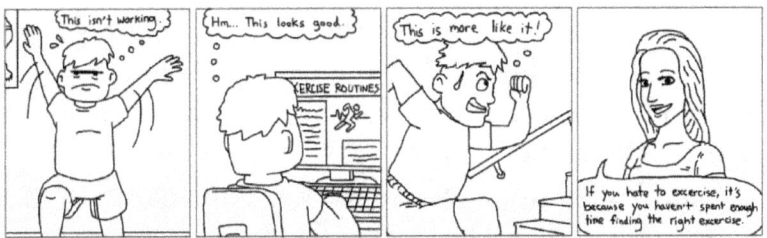

Exercise is a vital part of staying both mentally and physically healthy. Here are some questions to help you determine how much you know about exercise.

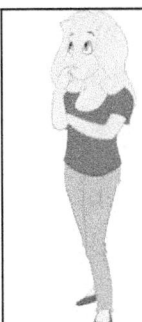

Q1: Have you tried a new exercise in the last 6 months?

Q2: Do you know how different exercises compare in calories burned?

Q3: Do you have at least 2-3 fun exercises that you've done in the last 6 months?

A person may expect that a book about thinking skinny has a long chapter on exercise. This book instead will focus around one idea on exercise. That idea is that the fun involved is way more important than the calories lost. A fun exercise is more likely to be repeated than a hard one.

Building a regular exercise routine takes a price. Many of us are fearful of that price. However, we are paying the price right now, by reading this book full of tips. Learning these tips is an excellent way to start moving forward.

We may not now the full path we are heading, but the bright future ahead is promising. We know that our nagging apprehension in our health has led to this moment. We know that we are no longer in the stone age where food is a scarcity. We know that our lives are busy and that technology gets more complicated by the day. What we may not know, is that working out can be not only fun, but a source of relaxation.

Often a workout routine, once in place, will help a person relax from their day. Not only do they burn off calories, but they also burn off stress. Why is that? Because they enjoy their workouts and have fun with them. Many times skinny people will have an endorphin rush when working out. We know this circumstance as "runners high". This mental space is where skinny people like to be when working out. The amount of calories is not important, the fun involved is important.

When a skinny person doesn't workout for several days, they start to feel dirty or not right. Working out is a way of cleansing and feeling better.

This chapter will focus on many workout suggestions. The hope is that after wards a few of these will be worth trying out. However, even if none of these suggestions hit home, the hope is that the curiosity of finding a fun exercise will take root.

Making working out more interesting

Exercise can shift from exciting to boring with repetition. Here are several simple but effective ideas to make any exercise routine more fun. These can also be used to help build a new set of exercises.

Change Exercises Regularly

Don't wait to get bored. Take a step towards being preventative and change the routine before it gets boring. As previously stated, there are many exercise ideas out there. Many apps and pod casts focus around new in-home and outside exercises that can be done. Furthermore, many exercises target specific muscle groups, which can lead to new challenge. Some require a level of commitment to earn a shirt or get some kind of trophy. This gamification of working out can also help keep exercise fun.

Find a Pro

In Think Like a Skinny Person, most of these ideas came from other people. They are compiled from these experts and presented here. Using this same technique can help build new exercise fun. Finding a professional trainer at a gym or privately can open up an avenue to ask questions. Furthermore, these people have spent a lot of time finding and perfecting exercise. They make the ideal knowledge targets when first learning about exercise. While learning what works for you is important, learning another person's journey can help shed some additional light on your own journey.

Get Geeky

Smart phones and tablets make working out amazing. Not only are there many working out applications available, there are also a lot of media to be consumed. For example, having a workout station can help inspire a person to push hard on their routine. Being able to catch up on a TV program may make exercise more fun. Reading a book, via an audio book, may also be a fantastic way to make exercise more fun. Not only do these ideas help make working out the body more fun, but they also help workout the brain. Many devices even have calorie and workout trackers. Some smart phones and tablets even have external devices they can talk to that will help track progress. For example, a blue tooth heat rate monitor that syncs with your phone and tells you how well you did versus yesterday. Or an application that syncs with your phone to help publish a "I ran here" map on social media. Technology is a fantastic way to enhance any workout.

Ready to go

Many experts put together home workouts for people to try. These are presented to people through a series of videos or workbooks. A new trend with these training systems is to help build the gamification. This trend includes providing free t-shirts and other gifts, if the user reaches a specific goal. The hope is that the user will provide before/after shots. These systems are usually pretty good, because they build a community around the exercise routines. These small communities help inspire others and help show how to successfully complete these exercise routines.

Get social

A great thing about the Internet is not how isolated people can become, but how it connects all of us. There are many websites that will allow people to find each. Some of these websites, like Meetup.com, help people who have similar interests get together. This can include people who like to hike or do other fun exercise routines. Becoming social around exercise is a great way to be inspired to do more. Not only is a person exercising their body, but they are also getting social time in. To extraverts, this is an ideal combination and a great way to make exercise fun. Many gyms also have a variety of social classes to try out. The idea is that a person can join a gym and then try out a bunch of different types of exercise. With any luck, they will find an exercise they really enjoy and will continue going to the gym.

Gear up

This suggestion is close to the get geeky suggestion, but with one difference. Many times people who gear up for exercise also get specific clothing or shoes. This can be an expensive way to be inspired to exercise, but it can be a great way to make it more fun. Having a special pair of workout shoes, or a fun water bottle, can make exercising more interesting.

Hidden Pockets of Time

One unique idea with making exercise fun is to find different times to exercise. Many times we get in the same time slot routine, which can get boring. If we change these time lines to be early morning or late at night, they may feel interesting and unique. Perhaps we get a different vision of the gym we belong to. Perhaps the usual people we see during our runs are different. Maybe it just feels better to get the workout done first thing. Perhaps we sleep better by getting the workout done late at night. Whatever the time line, changing the specific timing of exercising can be a way to spice working out up.

Goals

This technique fits very well into gearing up and getting geeky. Set a fitness goal to try and work towards. Perhaps this goal is distance ran or calories burned. When the goal is reached, reward yourself with something fun. Getting something fun that will help working out (such as new gear or a new geeky device) is ideal. Not only will a person be inspired once, but twice. First when working toward getting the reward. The second time when trying out the reward.

Hopefully these suggestions will make any exercise routine more fun. By staying flexible, we can build a momentum towards having more fun in our workouts. The more fun that is had, the better. Building fun is an ideal path towards making working out and weight loss a regular routine.

Outdoor Exercise Ideas

In the previous part we discussed ways to make exercise more fun. Here are some external, out of the house, exercise ideas that may work well. Ideally, the hunt should be on for finding the exercise. Finding fun exercise is one of the best things a person can do for themselves.

Running

One popular idea is to try running. This idea is much more cost effective over a gym. There is also a huge community of runners and many geeky devices to be tried out. These devices can track the location, steps taken, heart rate, calories burned, and much more. Running is a great way to become healthy and discover new stuff. Furthermore, the term "runners high" is not a made up phenomenon. Runners do have endorphins hit their brain when they have gone for long enough.

Sports

Many of us will never be professional athletes. However, that is not a good reason to avoid playing sports. People often enjoy coming together and playing a game of dodge ball, volleyball, softball, and even capture the flag. These sports may not be serious, but the amount of fun to be had is off the charts. These sports help a person go out and have fun, while not even noticing they are working out.

Hiking

Going on a hike is a great external activity to have fun. People can have fun exploring and playing in the outdoors while also getting fresh air. One of the best things about hiking is that there are so many different trails to try out. Many trails even have little amenities to go with them. Some trails may have a lake and fishing. Other trails have fantastic views and great places to take photographs. Some trails are very dog friendly. Hiking is also a great way to spend some quality one-on-one time with a loved one. Not only will hiking provide an excellent workout, but they also provide a way to spark conversation and have that intimate moment.

Biking

Another common activity to do outside is biking. This practice is much like running, but with less wear on the joints. Biking allows a person to discover their neighborhood without much effort. Many bike rides can also include pets and family, which can help make the experience a great bonding time.

Walking the dog

A daily dog walk is a great way to keep your pup happy. This method is also a great way to get in some exercise. Furthermore, many people can walk their dog to a dog park, which helps wear out the dog even more. The only trouble with this particular exercise is if the weather is miserable out. However, dogs can be dried off after a rain storm, so getting out of the house may be worth getting soaked.

Geo-caching

This outdoor activity is gaining popularity quickly. With geo-caching, a person uses a GPS to find a treasure. They then leave a small treasure for the next person. The great thing about geo-caching is that the activity doesn't feel like exercise. Furthermore more, geo-caching allows a person to play with new gadgets. However, all that is needed to get started is a smart phone with GPS, which most smart phones now have. That makes geo-caching more cost effective, since many people already have the equipment required. Geo-caching can be done with adults or children, which makes the experience a great way to bond with loved ones.

Indoor Exercise Ideas

Not all exercises are outside. Some exercises can be done regardless of weather. Many of these activities are also low cost or free. Here are several indoor exercises that may work well.

Gyms

Many people start here with this obvious choice. Many gyms have traditional equipment to help with cardiovascular or weight lifting. However, some may have extra courts, workout classes, and leagues to enjoy. These include basketball and racquetball courts, yoga, swimming, tennis, soccer, and many other types of exercise. Finding a gym with these features also means finding people drawn to those features. This idea can be great for being social while exercising.

Video Game Workouts

In the past video games were always associated with not working out. However, many modern consoles have options to complete a workout while also having fun. These low cost video games allow a person to try out a variety of movements to complete an objective. Many video game consoles have dancing options. Some video game consoles have action/adventure games that require exercise. Some video game consoles have games that require white water rafting or being a ninja. There are many different games to be tried out that can lead to fantastic workouts. Furthermore, these games build up points which allow a person to challenge their friends and family. These games also provide a way to dance to a favorite song and have fun.

Home Exercise Machines

These are much like machines a gym, but with the convenience of being located in the home. These machines can be ideal for a person who wants to fit in a quick workout. They also are ideal for those trying to save on gym membership or are wanting to watch a favorite TV program. A great thing about having this available is that weather is no longer an excuse to not workout. Even if the weather is snowing outside or raining outside, the exercise equipment is warm and ready to be used.

Shopping

Shopping is another idea to get up and walk around. This one is a bit more dangerous though, as many malls have random food courts and food vendors. Another idea is to walk around a book store reading what you want. These books help increase knowledge while also making exercise interesting. Gift stores and home decorating stores are also great places to walk around. These types of stores offer many things to look at and interact with, which can increase the amount you are walking around.

Indoor Mini-Golf

Many places have indoor mini-golf. These are great ways to have fun and walk around. Many times indoor golf serves as an ideal place to take a date. That is because the nature of mini-golf is to laugh at yourself and have fun. Not only does this activity help you bond with people, but it also helps burn a few calories.

Indoor Rock Climbing

Indoor rock climbing may work a bit better for those in great shape. With this venture, a person subscribes to a facility, much like a gym. In fact, many gyms now include some soft of indoor rock climbing. Each place provides both the proper safety equipment and training. Many of these places will also come with special classes designed to get more out of the sport. This activity is a great way to challenge yourself and burn a lot of calories.

Indoor Running

Many gyms and facilities have an indoor track to run on. These are fantastic ways to burn calories without having to worry about weather. Many people prefer to try out time trials with these tracks. Challenging yourself to do a little better each time is a great way to stay motivated. Furthermore, these indoor tracks can help a person stay connected. By having friends beside you while running, conversations and connections can be had.

The trick with working out as a skinny person is in finding a fun workout routine. Not only is finding fun important, but it can be a great way to relieve daily stress. Perhaps this stress relief is through the release of endorphins during runners high. Perhaps this stress relief is talking to someone while working out. Whatever the case may be, skinny people tend to feel like working out re-aligns or "cleans" them. Not only does the working out help them stay fit, it also helps with their daily mental attitude. The purpose of working out is not so much of weight loss to a skinny person, but rather releasing tension.

PART FIVE

Cooking

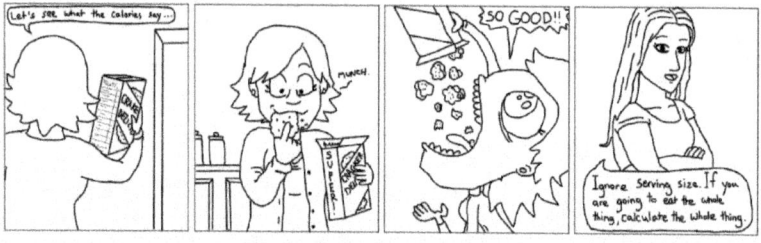

Cooking requires knowing your ingredients. Skinny people not only know about ingredients but actively seek out to learn more. Here are some questions to test your curiosity:

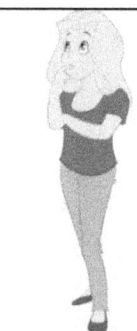

Q1: When was the last time you compared nutrition labels?

Q2: Have you shopped at a farmers market or specialty store in the last 6 months?

Q3: When was the last time you cooked with a new ingredient?

Skinny people know that making a great meal doesn't have to mean buying it pre-made. Many skinny people delight in making their own meals. Not only does this food taste better, because of the quality of ingredients, but a skinny person has more control of the meal. They can simply decrease calories by cutting down on less healthy parts of the meal. Furthermore, they can add in what they want to make the meal better.

The trick that many skinny people use is how they view food preparation. For many, there is dread around cooking. Skinny people perceive a certain joy in building their meal. They view this is as an exciting project, a challenge, that has great benefits. Others come up with excuses on why not to cook. Those excuses include skill, confidence, boredom, and cleaning up. Here are different perspectives on each of those excuses.

Skill can be easily corrected with a few cooking classes. Furthermore, there are many books aimed at cooking novices. Some of these books help cover the basic terminology and techniques that can be used elsewhere. The best way to build up a level of skill in cooking is to cook. Not everything will taste fantastic, but knowing what works and doesn't is a way of improving.

Another excuse is confidence. Many people host dinner parties for their family and friends. They are worried that their talents are not enough to please their guests. The key to defeating this lack of confidence is to be prepared. Planning the menu carefully can regain a sense of control. Furthermore, having spare ingredients, spare time, and a backup plan can help a person move forward with preparation.

Boredom is a common excuse among those who would cook. The solution to this is exceedingly simple - find a challenging dish. If a person is used to making homemade pasta, have them try cooking Thai or Indian. If they dislike those types of dishes, have them try unique pasta dishes or use "pasta like" substances. Furthermore, trying out different spices and seasonings can help bring new discovery to old dishes. There is always more to learn when discovering cooking.

Finally, there is the cleanup from cooking. Many dread cooking because of the cleanup. However, many couples get past this with a simple trick: one cooks and the other cleans. Another idea is to identify why a person hates cleaning. If it is the closeness of eating and cleaning, perhaps a quick rinse after eating, followed by a full clean later. If they hate scrubbing hard against the plates, perhaps cleaning the dishes right after eating. Perhaps a person hates to eat knowing they will have to work later. Maybe a compromise can be done to clean the pots and pans before eating. This can be done by chilling and re-heating the food. Furthermore, paper plates can reduce the amount of cleaning afterwards. Understanding why a person hates to clean is the first step in understanding how to defeat this behavior.

Cooking is a one-on-one experience

Skinny people are focused with establishing a good relationship with food. Part of this relationship is understanding the components of food. For some, they will look at the nutrition of each ingredient to see if it falls within their guidelines. Other skinny people will look at the cost of each individual ingredient, or the cost of a serving of the food. Finally, other people will look at the fun of a cooking a dish. In each of these circumstances, a skinny person is looking at the individual ingredients to see how they feel about them. The more they enjoy those ingredients, and have confidence in using them, the more likely they will become staples.

To start this food relationship, many skinny people will go on a discovery of food. This discovery may start with a Google search or a grocery store visit. Either way they look at the ingredient and take it through a number of checklists. If they feel the ingredient will work with their diets, they will give it a try.

The same is true for trying out and discovering individual spices. Many home cooks know a dish fairly well and are looking to enhance that dish. Getting a specific spice that does that, while maintaining the required dietary restrictions can be fantastic. The world is full of unique spices, so there are always new ways to build food combinations.

Finally, a skinny person will investigate the different cooking techniques. They know that a particular food may work well and give them bragging rights. Not only will new cooking techniques build up their skills, but their social standing as well.

Cooking is also a social experience

Discovering new ingredients, spices, and cooking techniques are not the only reason skinny people cook. They also embrace the social aspect of building food. These skinny people enjoy the idea that their efforts will bring joy and pleasure to those around them. Many cultures use cooking and eating as reasons to be social and connect with those around you.

One of the best examples of this is during the holidays. Baking special holiday treats is one way a person can show they care for another. Many people look forward to these unique treats. This natural give and take helps build social connection between two groups of people.

Some baking includes building edible decorations. Many times a person will build dishes that celebrate that unique holiday. For example, fruit in the shape of a flag for independence day or Frankenstein cookies for Halloween. These unique foods can serve as not only treats, but edible decorations.

Holidays are not the only time skinny people enjoy making food. Semi-unique events, such as birthdays, barbecues, and romantic evenings are all reasons to make food. Making food for a group of family and friends is a great way to contribute to a gathering. They know that making fantastic food can really liven up the party. Skinny people also know that spending a night in doing some romantic cooking can spice things up. Not only does this show compassion, cooking also shows desire. Compassion is shown by paying attention to a person's likes and dislikes. Desire can be added into the mix by cooking together. Many men and women find a partner that cooks to be irresistible.

Skinny people cook and bake for a variety of reasons. The biggest among those is to continue establishing a healthy relationship with food. By building a great relationship with food, guilt and ill effects are minimized. Skinny people know that one of the main keys to their health is in establishing healthy staples to eat regularly.

PART SIX

Conclusion

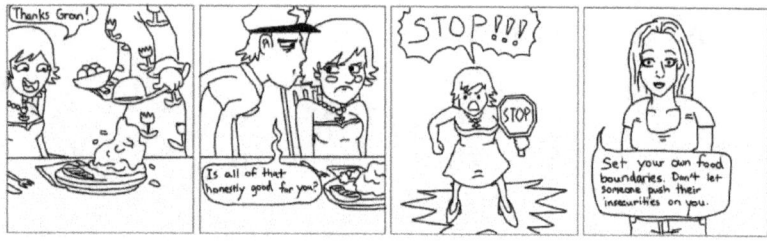

Beware of people dictating your relationship with food! Food pushers and food police can easily ruin your diet. Even this book should be met with skepticism. Go out and seek your balance!

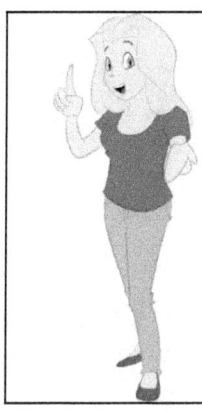

Thank you for reading this book!

Hopefully you enjoyed it. If you did not like this book, please let me know.

(james@thinklikeaskinnyperson.com)

If you enjoyed the style of this book,
I also have the website up full of more tips:
www.thinklikeaskinnyperson.com

Thanks again!

James